# Total Health Upgrade

## Peak Performance for Executives and Professionals

DR. BRUCE EICHELBERGER, OMD

# DEDICATION

To all my patients for the past 42 years. Thank you for all that you've taught me about the resilience of human beings and their ability to heal. Thank you also to my teachers who have shared their knowledge, wisdom and experience, especially when I needed it most.

# CONTENTS

# ACKNOWLEDGMENTS

My gratitude goes to so many that I cannot name all of them here. I am especially grateful to Master Share K. Lew, who helped me understand how to directly perceive the state of someone's health. Also to Dr. Robert Anderson, who took that understanding to a whole new level. William Wolcott, who constantly reminded me that humans are designed to work perfectly and that any symptom can come from any cause. Neil Gumenick, who helped me understand more deeply how every level of human experience is connected to health and healing. Finally, Robert Middleton, who encouraged me to see that the world was ready to receive this information

# 1. WHY DON'T YOU FEEL BETTER?

There is an epidemic going on that nobody is talking about. About 80% of the population has it.

What is it? I call it, "Unwell Syndrome."

How do you know you have it? One way is that you just don't feel right. Another is that you go to your doctor and after running a few tests, she pronounces that there is nothing wrong. "Try and relax more," she says. Or maybe she tells you to "eat better."

Yeah, right.

You know when you feel your best and when you don't. Unfortunately, the modern, disease-based medical model doesn't always have a way to get you back on track.

Sure, you can use over-the-counter remedies. After all, it's a multi-billion dollar industry, so obviously lots of people use them. They are mostly natural. And sometimes they do just what they promise. But sometimes they don't. Even if it worked for your best friend, it might not work for you. Are you willing to play hit or miss with your health?

So what's the alternative?

There is a secret out there you should know. That is that your body is designed to work perfectly. It has amazing healing and repair capabilities. It can adapt to an astounding number of conditions. And it can reach higher levels of health than you might now imagine.

This book is designed to help you get to those higher levels. I know that seems like a tall order. And you should know it will take some action on your part to get there. But the effort will be worth it.

The purpose of this book is to cut to the chase and give you a real chance to see improvements. You will not find complex theories. And you will not find impossible to follow regimens. What you will find are the facts. They are based on over 40 years of working with patients to help them achieve higher-level health.

This book is divided into 6 chapters. Chapter 2 gives you an overview of why chronic disease happens. Chapter 3 offers natural ways to deal with symptoms. Chapter 4 talks about how to fix deeper causes of symptoms. Chapter 5 gives you information to help you repair damage caused over time. Finally, the sixth chapter outlines an ideal program of restoring your health.

I encourage you to take these ideas seriously. With a bit of knowledge and noticing the outcomes, you will see improvements before you know it.

## 2. THE IRONY OF AGING

As you age, you are (hopefully) becoming wiser. You have a great deal more experience. The things you know, you generally know very well.

The irony is that aging also brings signs of decline. Less energy. More aches and pains. A harder time focusing as well as you used to.

There are lots of reasons for this. This book won't spend a lot of time going over the reasons. You will learn some of them along the way, but mostly you will know about them so you will know how to correct them.

Decline isn't mandatory. You know this if you look around you. Although you certainly know people who are less healthy than they used to be, you can also see examples of people who are thriving. It's those people we all want to emulate.

But how do these people get this way? Obviously genetics plays a role. And their life history. And, of course, their lifestyle.

Although we can't take in their genetics or replicate their life history, we can learn things from their lifestyle. But that isn't the only factor for reaching excellent health.

Why? Because the body is enormously complex. And because the body is so complex, it isn't possible to fix one small part without affecting all of the others. That makes simple, one-shot remedies impractical. There are too many potential side effects to have that work well.

An easier, and more effective way to deal with this complexity is by looking at the inputs and outputs to and from the body.

Why does this work? It's because it reduces the number of things you need to pay attention to. And that makes the enormous complexity of human health easier to deal with.

The following diagram gives you an idea of what that looks like:

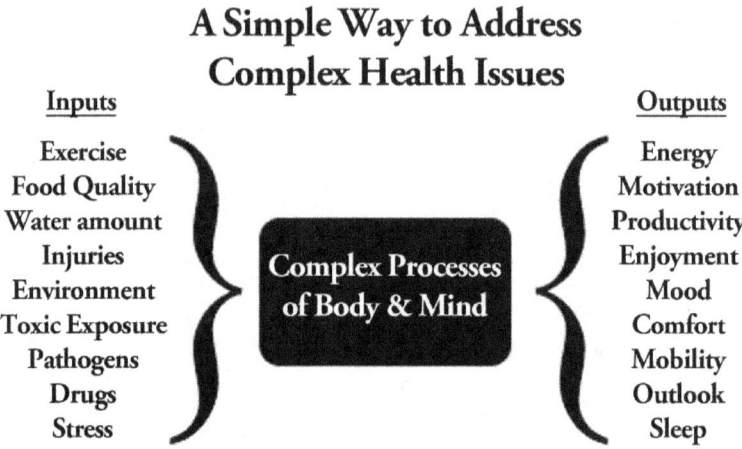

## A Simple Way to Address Complex Health Issues

**Inputs**

Exercise
Food Quality
Water amount
Injuries
Environment
Toxic Exposure
Pathogens
Drugs
Stress

**Complex Processes of Body & Mind**

**Outputs**

Energy
Motivation
Productivity
Enjoyment
Mood
Comfort
Mobility
Outlook
Sleep

By making adjustments to inputs, we can monitor how they affect you by watching the outputs. Simple, isn't it?

Of course on the inside many things are going on. The Total Health Upgrade Program focuses on inputs and outputs, but it is also useful to know the kinds of changes that can happen. To that end, here is a list of the most important internal factors that contribute to a decline in health:

- **Inflammation** – this is the body's attempt to fight infection and promote healing. For something like a cut or bruise, this is a good thing. But if you have inflammation all the time, something is wrong. And masking the symptoms with pain relievers never fixes the real problem. Over time this damages your health in multiple ways.

- **Changes in DNA** – this especially refers to the length of your telomeres. Telomeres are the part of your DNA that protects its ability to replicate and create new proteins. When these shorten over time, it reduces your ability to bounce back from injury and disease.

- **Free radicals and oxidative damage caused by them** – these are one of the primary causes of aging. They are highly reactive. When there are too many of them, they interfere with proteins, fatty acids and even your DNA.

- **Exposure to toxins** – toxins are everywhere in modern life. They exist in building materials, foods, clothing, cleaning products and the air you breathe.

- **Maillard reactions and AGEs** – no, a Maillard is not a duck. Rather it refers to the action of cooking down proteins and sugars to create a caramel-like substance in the body. This substance is called Advanced Glycation End-products (AGEs). As you might imagine, if you have caramel in your cells, they can't function right.

- **Hormone imbalances** – as you age, your hormone levels change. The most commonly talked about one is women who go through menopause. But men also have hormone changes as they age. And stress can be a major factor in reducing quality of life, including sex drive.

- **Brain chemistry imbalances** – anxiety, depression, fatigue, irritability and chronic sadness are all symptoms that are closely related to brain chemistry. Unfortunately, the mainstream drugs used to treat these conditions often come with a long list of side effects. And they are often hard to stop taking.

- **Stress and trauma** – both emotional and physical stress can cause long-term stress in your body.

- **Beliefs and attitudes** – if you've ever known someone who is always negative, you can see how it affects their quality of life. Modern research has discovered that unproductive beliefs trigger almost immediate negative changes in the body.

- **Activity level** – both mental and physical activity are important for quality of life. Both are good examples of the maxim, "use it or lose it."

- **Muscle loss** – if you don't use your muscles, you will eventually lose muscle mass. And over time, this causes secondary problems. Doing daily activities becomes harder. Falls and other accidents become more common.

- **Decreased mitochondria function** – mitochondria are the energy generators in every cell in your body. Over time they can lose efficiency. This can lead to fatigue and low motivation.

That's some list, isn't it? Fortunately, you don't have to think about every one of these issues. There are some simple things you can do that will improve all of them at once. That's why we will be focusing on inputs and outputs.

Don't worry if you haven't heard of some of these. By the time you are done reading, you will have the information you need to reverse the effects of declining health.

# 3. HOW TO ADDRESS SYMPTOMS NATURALLY

To rebuild your health requires correcting the deep, underlying causes of illness. But that doesn't always relieve your symptoms quickly. Sometimes you want symptomatic relief right away.

That's what this chapter is about. But before offering the details, I want to be very clear about one thing. The whole point of this book is to give you the tools to be able to correct the underlying issues. **If you want real, lasting results, please don't only rely on relieving symptoms.**

Okay?

Symptomatic relief is the specialty of allopathic medicine. This is what most modern medical doctors practice. I call it the "have this problem, take this pill" approach. And you can do the same type of thing with natural remedies that most prescription drugs do. In other words, you can often find remedies that will help manage symptoms. But taken this way, even natural remedies can miss getting to the root of the problem.

In addition, natural remedies can have the same issues that over-the-counter medicines and prescription drugs have. They can mask symptoms. They can become less effective over time. You might have to take more to get the same result.

That being said, here are some of the best natural ways to address chronic health symptoms:

## Low Energy and Poor Mental Focus

These are almost always a result of long-term, deeper issues. As a result, there are not very many ways to reliably fix these at the symptom level. At best, symptomatic solutions get you by, but there is a price to pay.

The obvious choice, coffee, will address both of these. But at best it gets you by. It won't correct the real issues. However, if you need it to help your energy, focus and clarity while fixing the deeper issues, by all means use it.

You can get additional temporary relief with the following natural remedies:

- **Vitamin B12** – best take as a lozenge or spray under the tongue. That's because it is harder to absorb in your stomach. Putting it directly under your tongue gets it straight into your blood stream.

- **Siberian Ginseng (Eleutherococcus)** – a good adaptogen for supporting energy and focus.

- **Rosemary** – more for mental focus and memory than energy. Generally safe in recommended amounts.

- **Gotu Kola** – this herb acts as a mild stimulant. If you are diabetic, note that it may raise blood sugar levels.

- **Ginkgo Biloba** – dilates blood vessels in the brain, allowing better blood flow. Caution if you are on blood thinners. Avoid taking if you are on antidepressants.

For any of these, start with a lower dose and gradually increase until you get the result you are looking for. Dosages will be on the bottle.

## Pain

Most pain has an inflammatory component to it. That's why people take aspirin and other over-the-counter anti-inflammatories. But there are side effects from these drugs. Here are the natural options.

### Enzymes

As you age, your body becomes less efficient at making enzymes. But when you have enough enzymes in your system, they can scavenge inflammation. That means they break down the inflammatory substances in your joints, muscles and organs.

Here is a list of useful enzymes for this purpose:

- **Bromelain** – an enzyme that comes from pineapple. It reduces swelling and inflammation. Some studies show it can be effective against arthritis pain and stiffness. It also has beneficial effects on digestion, breathing and circulation.

- **Papain** – from papayas. This enzyme helps break down proteins. Good for inflammation and swelling.

- **Chymotrypsin** – this enzyme is also good at digesting proteins. It is used medically to reduce inflammation and swelling. Made in the body, but can also be taken as a supplement.

- **Trypsin** – similar to chymotrypsin.

If you are taking enzymes to control inflammation, it is best not to take them with food. If you do, they will be used up breaking down the food and there will be less available for attacking inflammation.

Note that you can take more than one of these at a time. Online or at your local health food store, you can find enzyme combinations that contain more than one of these

### Natural Anti-inflammatories

In addition to enzymes, there are herbs and nutrients that are very helpful to support your body's efforts to reduce pain.

- **Omega-3 fatty acids** – EPA and DHA. The best forms of these are in fish oil or krill oil.

- **Ginger root** – fighting inflammation is only one of ginger's many health benefits. Use the fresh root (cooking or tea) or buy it in capsule form.

- **Curcumin** – a compound of the spice, turmeric. Best to use a specific extract of this rather than the spice when you want relief for inflammation. You can take up to a gram of the extract at a time.

- **Boswellia serrata** – also called Indian frankincense. Used for arthritis and other chronic inflammatory diseases. Sometimes used as an alternative to NSAIDs (aspirin, ibuprofen, Tylenol, etc.)

- **Feverfew** – this herb is most commonly used to reduce migraine headaches. There is some evidence it also reduces joint pain.

### Amino Acids

These are protein building blocks. The following are great for pain relief:

- **MSM** – this is the third-largest nutrient found in the human body. It is a sulfur-containing amino acid. It is especially helpful for joint pain.

- **DLPA** – prolongs the pain-relieving effect of your body's natural pain reliever, endorphins. Take 500 mg up to 4 times a day to start. You can gradually increase to 3,000 to 4,000 mg 4 times a day if needed. **Caution!** Do not use DLPA if you have phenylketonuria (PKU) or tardive dyskinesia. Your doctor would have told you if you had either of these.

## Self-care Techniques

There is no care like self-care. Pain often responds well to specific activities. There are potentially many of these, but here are some of the best. You will want to consult with your doctor before undergoing any of these techniques:

- **Exercise** – often pain is a result of lack of use of muscles and joints. Ironically, the pain often keeps a person from exercising. If you do decide to exercise when you have chronic pain, start slow. And make sure your doctor is okay with it. Be sure to notice if the exercise is increasing the pain or not. If it is, either stop or change the exercise you are doing.

- **Yoga** – generally more gentle than most exercise. It focuses on stretching and holding postures. This can really help reduce pain when done regularly.

- **Qigong** – a Chinese form of yoga, it is done in slow, gentle movements. Done correctly, these movements can increase your range of motion and decrease your pain levels.

Obviously you will need some instruction to do yoga and qigong. Books, videos on the internet, DVDs and classes are your best bets for this. And you don't have to get extreme with any of these. Even regular walking can make a huge difference. If you do decide to exercise, you might consider consulting a personal trainer who can help you get the most out of exercise without hurting yourself.

## Professional Care

In the worst case, you might need to see a professional to help manage pain symptoms while you are fixing the underlying issues. I recommend the following:

- **Massage** – relaxing and good for increasing circulation, especially to muscles.

- **Acupuncture** – excellent for pain relief, it also can correct the deeper underlying issues.

- **Chiropractic** – very helpful for back and neck pain.

- **Aston Patterning** – helps you realign your movement so that it is in harmony with your body. Pain often disappears almost like magic when you get everything working right.

- **Cranio-sacral Therapy** – more gentle and subtle than any of the other options.

These remedies and techniques will go a very long way towards the goal of relieving symptoms. But I will remind you again that if you want real, long-term results, you should correct the deeper causes of health issues. Read on to the next chapter for more on this.

DR. BRUCE EICHELBERGER

# 4. FINDING AND FIXING DEEPER CAUSES OF SYMPTOMS

Your body is complex.

For example, there are 50,000 biochemical reactions going on all the time. This is part of why drugs that affect just one or two of them can't fix the deeper problems. They are too focused on one thing to deal with all of the related processes going on in your body.

I like to compare taking high-powered drugs to shooting a high-powered rifle... at the ocean. Yes, it has a big impact at the moment. But the "ocean" of the other 49,999 biochemical reactions soon adapts around the impact.

This explains why drugs often become less effective over time. And it also explains the common experience of side effects. These aren't so much a problem of bad drug design as they are a reflection of your body's incredible ability to adapt. And the reason your body has to adapt is that these drugs don't fix what creates the symptoms in the first place. Only by fixing the underlying problem can you get rid of them for good.

## Deeper Healing in Two Steps

Simply put, there are only two things that need to be addressed to correct deep causes of disease. They are:

1. **Stop doing things that interfere with your body's natural functioning.** These are sometimes called "blocking factors." Since your body is designed to work perfectly, it makes sense to stop interfering with it.

2. **Start doing things that support your body's health and balance.** There are some very specific ways you can support health.

I told you it was simple. But of course, the devil is in the details. So let's get right to them.

## Step 1: Eliminate Blocking Factors Interfering with Your Body's Natural Functioning

First, you should know that your body has amazing abilities to neutralize things which interfere with normal, healthy functioning. If it didn't, humans would have died out a very long time ago.

That being said, in modern times you face far more blocking factors that ever in history. That means your ability to neutralize them is more likely to be overwhelmed.

As just one example of the proliferation of blocking factors, consider that 1,000 to 3,000 new chemicals are introduced into the environment every year. And this has been going on for the past 30 years! You can bet that most of these have not been tested for toxic potential.

What are some examples of blocking factors? Here's a short list:

- **Toxins in your food** – preservatives, coloring, flavor enhancers, etc.

- **Toxins in your environment** – building materials, pesticides, herbicides, cleaning solutions, chemicals in rugs and clothing designed to stop mold, etc.

- **Pathogens and parasites** – these include viruses, bacteria and mold

- **Food sensitivities** – the technical name for these is adverse food reactions. There are 4 levels of these, some of which are very hard to identify on your own.

- **Unnatural foods** – overly processed foods, genetically modified foods (GMO).

- **Drugs** – Both prescription and recreational. Any drug tends to change just one or a few biochemical reactions. That means it will likely have unintended interference with other body functions.

- **Physical trauma** – injuries, surgeries, over-use.

- **Mental and emotional stress** – relationship problems, work pressures, deadlines, money issues, especially if these occur over a long time.

How do you eliminate these? It helps if you know which of them are the biggest problems. To know what toxins are present requires testing. A doctor trained in functional medicine can run tests to determine this.

However, you can assume that your body has been assaulted by many or most of these blocking factors. And because of that there are steps you can take to deal with them.

For toxic exposure, you want to make sure that you reduce exposure to potential problems. Here are specific ways to handle this.

- **Breathe Pure Air** – Get air filters for your home. I recommend ionic air filters.

- **Drink Pure Water** – Use reverse osmosis water filters for drinking water.

- **Wash in Pure Water** – Install shower head filters on all showers to remove chlorine.

- **Reduce Toxic Soaps and Cleaners** – As much as possible, use natural cleaning products. This includes antibacterial soaps. The triclosan most of them contain can disrupt hormones and can also lead to resistant bacteria. Natural soap works just as well to kill germs.

- **Avoid Processed Foods** – That means most of those that come in a jar, a bottle, a can, a box or a package. And when you must eat some of these, check the ingredients. Anything you can't pronounce is a red flag. So is anything that is vague, like "natural flavoring."

- **Manage Your Stress** – When possible remove yourself from stressful situations. If that isn't possible, find ways to reduce the impact of them. Exercise, meditation, prayer, deep breathing and self-hypnosis are all helpful. Taking up an enjoyable hobby will also help.

- **Move Your Body** – Exercise, such as walking, swimming, yoga and qigong help maintain and restore normal function. As a bonus, exercise also supports your ability to think clearly.

- **Reduce Drug Exposure** – Both prescription and non-prescription. For prescription drugs, only do this with the guidance of your doctor. And only do this in either case while fixing deeper causes.

In addition to avoiding things, you can also support your body's ability to remove toxic materials. Self-care ways to do this include coffee enemas, intermittent fasting and herbal cleanses.

There is also a particular product that is designed to help your body remove most toxins. It is called D-Toxol. You can do an internet search to find where to buy this.

If you decide to use D-Toxol, I recommend you start with a low amount until you see if it is clearing out toxins too fast or not. If you feel fine after a few days, gradually increase the dose up to the amount listed on the label.

When you are ready to find out more, find a doctor versed in functional medicine. He or she will test for exposure to toxins and pathogens. You will also get tested to find out the efficiency of your ability to remove toxins. Both are crucial to supporting your health.

## Step 2: Do Things to Actively Support Your Health

It isn't enough to stop doing those things that interfere with your body's natural functions. You also have to actively support your health.

Even if you think you know about some of these techniques, it is worth looking this list over. You might learn something new.

### Improve Your Diet

By this I mean two things. The first has to do with food sensitivities. See more on this aspect in Step 1 above.

The second is eating primarily the specific high-energy foods your body need. This is equally important.

But how do you figure out what these foods are? Do you look at the government's food pyramid? No. Definitely not.

The best way I've run across over the past 40 years is called Metabolic Typing® (MT). Over the past 40 or so years this system has been refined and developed.

Without going into great detail, MT recognizes that each person is unique. Think about it – nobody looks or acts the same on the outside. Why would we think our food requirements are all exactly the same? It turns out they aren't.

The process requires filling out a fairly extensive questionnaire. There are about 160 questions.

The results do several things. First, they give you a list of foods color-coded based on how they affect your metabolism. This is invaluable information. By sticking to foods listed as ideal for you, you will notice improvement in your health.

Second, you will understand how to dial-in the ideal ratios of fats, proteins and carbohydrates. This is the key to making the list completely yours.

How do you go about taking this test? There are several ways. The simplest is to buy the book, "The Metabolic Typing Diet" by William Wolcott and Trish Fahey. It has some good information in it and a basic, 64-question test.

Although the test in the book will give you some general results, they aren't as fine-tuned as other ways to take the test.

The second way to take the test is online. The web address is www.MetabolicTypingOnline.com. This test is essentially the same as the one I send my patients to.

The downside to this approach is that you don't have personal guidance and support in the process. But if you are motivated and focused, it can be a great way to get started.

The third way to do MT testing is with a Certified Metabolic® Typing Advisor (CMTA). You can find people all over the world trained in this approach. And because the test is done online, the person you work with doesn't even have to be in the same town as you are. I've worked with patients as far away as Kazakhstan. Using email and Skype, this is entirely possible.

### Address Functional Processes

This refers to the basic actions your body needs to perform to be healthy. It is the realm of Functional Medicine.

What areas are best focused on?

- **Digestive efficiency** – your ability to digest and assimilate nutrients, especially protein.

- **Detoxification capacity** – your ability to eliminate poisons through your liver, lungs, skin, kidneys and intestines.

- **Oxidative stress** – how well you neutralize free radicals.

- **Adrenal fatigue** – how well you deal with and recover from stress.

Can you do some of this on your own? Possibly.

For example, you can take digestive enzymes and digestive hydrochloric acid to support your digestion. You can also take antioxidants in supplement form. See more about these options in Chapter 5.

You might also want to support your detoxification capacity. The best way to do this, as mentioned previously, is with D-Toxol.

You can get a generalized adrenal support supplement. This will have adaptogen herbs in it. Siberian ginseng, rhodiola, ashwaganda, reishi mushrooms and schizandra are among the herbs you will find in these formulas. Some will also have B vitamins and other nutrients.

If you want a more focused approach, which will save you time and avoid the need to do everything yourself, find a doctor who practices Functional Medicine.

## Rebalance Structure and Energy Flow

If you use your body incorrectly, by habit or as a result of injury, it adds stress to your system. It also interferes with the flow of vital energy that keeps your body working well. By correcting these problems, you take away the need for your body to compensate and adapt to this stress.

Here are the ways you can accomplish this:

- **Exercise** – especially strength-building exercises. These can be body-weight types of exercise (pushups, deep knee bends, etc.) They can also be done with weights. I very highly recommend you work with a trainer if you are at all unfamiliar with doing this type of exercise. It will save you time, give you better results, and reduce the chance of injury. As always, clear this with your doctor.

- **Yoga** – a time-tested practice that strengthens and stretches your body. Again, find some way to get guidance. At the least, use a video. The idea option is to take a class or get one-to-one training.

- **Stretching** – simple stretching can go a long way towards improving your overall physical function. At the very least, get up from sitting at least every 30 minutes and move around. If you can gently stretch when you do this, it will be better.

- **Qigong** – this is a form of working with vital energy in your body. The exercises are typically gentle and suitable for people of any age and fitness. As with the other choices in this section, getting instruction will make sure you get the most benefit from your practice.

There are also professional services that will help you get your body back into optimal functioning. Here is a list of my favorites:

- **Acupuncture** – good for much more than just relieving symptoms. In particular, Classical Five Element Acupuncture is outstanding for correcting many types of imbalance in the body, mind and spirit. It is a complete system of medicine in and of itself.

- **Chiropractic** – a well-trained and experienced chiropractor will not only focus on realigning your spine, he or she will also pay attention to functional aspects of healing.

- **Aston Patterning** – this form of body work identifies structural misalignments and corrects them. In addition, you will learn how to use your body in ways that reduce tension and increase efficiency. Very highly recommended.

- **Massage** – a good massage helps your body relax, improves circulation and relieves stress. It also gives you a chance to relax and let go for an hour.

- **Cranio-sacral Therapy** – a gentle way to help your nervous system by reducing trauma and restoring balance. When done by an experienced practitioner, this subtle work goes deep and corrects fundamental imbalances.

## Manage Stress More Effectively

Stress is a big deal. Sometimes patients come into my practice and talk about their stress as if it were nothing. Their symptoms say otherwise.

I like to compare ongoing stress to getting hit by a bus. The main difference is the time it takes. A bus hits you all at once. Stress hits you over time. But the cumulative effect is very similar.

That means managing your stress is crucial for upgrading your health.

Ways to accomplish stress reduction:

- **Exercise** – funny how this one keeps coming up. And yes, exercise is an outstanding way to help manage stress. It gives you the opportunity to release pent-up energy and emotions. As a bonus, by taking you out of your normal routine, exercise can often be an aid to problem solving.

- **Meditation & prayer** – both are excellent for helping manage stress. Part of their effectiveness comes from focusing on something bigger than yourself. They help put your stresses into a better perspective.

- **Deep breathing** – sounds too simple, doesn't it? But research shows that deep, abdominal breathing triggers what is called "the relaxation response." What could be better when you are dealing with stress?

- **Self-hypnosis** – with a little training and some practice, you can use self-hypnosis to make deep changes. The ability to manage your own mental and emotional processes is very empowering!

- **Counseling** – if you still have a hard time managing stress, it's a good idea to find someone who can help you through it. It might be a therapist, a priest or rabbi or just a good friend who can listen.

# 5. REPAIRING DAMAGE AND REBUILDING HEALTH

Once you have managed symptoms and corrected the underlying causes, all that is left is to repair the damage that has already happened.

You will notice that a number of these approaches are similar to recommendations made in the previous chapter about fixing the underlying problems. The duplicates happen because they not only fix the imbalance, they also help rebuild health.

First of all, you want to make sure that you are supporting you overall health. That means two things – eating according to your unique metabolic needs and supplementing your diet with natural nutrients. As mentioned in Chapter 3, Metabolic Typing® (MT) is the best way to determine your ideal foods. If you want to go back and look at that section again, click here.

If you haven't done the MT testing, then you should look for a good quality multiple vitamin with minerals. If you have done the testing, you will have received an individualized list of optimal supplements for your type. Get them and take them.

For specific issues, here are some excellent ways to repair the damage and rebuild your health.

## Repairing Damaged Tissues

Inflammation and oxidation often leave behind tissue damage. This comes in two forms, fibrosis and connective tissue damage.

For fibrosis (tissue damage outside of joints), proteolytic enzymes work very well. These include:

- **Serrapeptase** – from the gut bacteria of silkworms. This enzyme reduces swelling and inflammation. It also stops certain types of pain. In addition, it helps break down fibrin. Fibrin is part of what clogs arteries. Breaking it down can help open up circulation.

- **Nattokinase** – a fermented soy derivative. If you use this, make sure it is made from organic soy. Not only breaks down fibrosis, but also lowers cholesterol.

- **Bromelain** – from pineapple. You learned about this in Chapter 2. Also excellent for inflammation and swelling.

- **Papain** – from papaya. Also from Chapter 2. Also an excellent way to reduce inflammation and swelling.

For joint damage, here are some good choices:

- **Glucosamine & chondroitin** – the natural building blocks for cartilage. Helps repair joint damage. Don't use glucosamine if you are allergic to shellfish.

- **Hyaluronic acid** – naturally concentrated in connective tissues and the eyes. When taken as a supplement, it can help restore joints and prevent against cartilage breakdown.

- **SAMe** – an amino acid. Found in every cell in the body. Relieves pain and swelling, but also helps rebuild cartilage. It can also relieve depression. That means if you are taking an anti-depressant medication, you should avoid it, or at least work with your doctor when taking it.

## Repair Adrenal Fatigue

Your adrenals are your organs of survival. Think about the idea of adrenalin. When you need to get something done in an emergency, you call on your adrenals. They are the source of your "fight or flight" response.

But they aren't designed to be in survival mode all the time. If you experience chronic stress, your adrenals are working too hard. As a result, they become less efficient over time.

One sign this is happening is if you are tired all the time or especially at certain times of the day. But there are many other signs as well. The health of your adrenals affects almost every other part of your body.

The following page shows an illustration of what can be affected if your adrenals are not healthy:

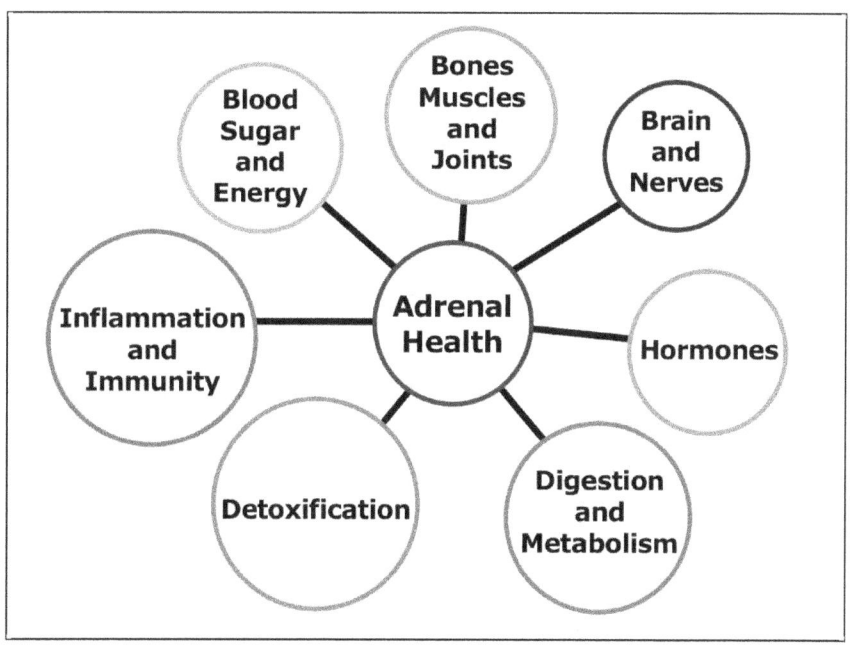

Chronic health issues and stress deplete adrenal reserves over time. This ends up depleting hormones essential to quality of life.

To manage this on your own, you can consider taking a general adrenal supplement. There is more information on this in Chapter 4.

If you want support dealing with this, a doctor trained in Functional Medicine can help. You will take a saliva test. By taking saliva samples multiple times over the course of a day, the degree and pattern of adrenal fatigue shows up. Your doctor will recommend a course a treatment specific to the degree and pattern of your symptoms.

## Support Detoxification Pathways

As mentioned before, the supplement D-Toxol is excellent for removing toxins of all kinds. However some people can release these poisons too quickly, causing a detox reaction. If you are taking this supplement, you can also take a supplement called Methyldote. It completely eliminates negative reactions to D-Toxol.

## Prevent Further Oxidative Damage

Taking supplements to repair damage caused by oxidative free radicals (see above) is an excellent step. But you also want to take steps to prevent further damage.

Why do you need to do this? Because your body is constantly making free radicals. These are the result of basic processes like breathing and eating. These free radicals cause oxidative stress when there are too many of them for your body to manage well. Many physicians feel these are a major contributor to aging. There is evidence that they also contribute to cancer.

How does your body manage free radicals? With antioxidants. That's why having the right amount of them is so important.

So what can you do to have the right amount?

Exercise goes a long way. So does not smoking. And the old standby, eating well, is high on the list as well. In this case, it means not eating processed foods, fried foods and bad fats. It does mean eating fresh, whole fruits and vegetables.

You can also get supplement formulas with a number of antioxidants included. Here is a list of what to look for:

- **Beta carotene** – the precursor for vitamin A.

- **Vitamins C and E** – both crucial for many body processes. Look for naturally sourced vitamin C. Also, don't use just simple vitamin E (alpha tocopherol). Find a supplement with all 4 tocopherols and all 4 tocotrienols.

- **N-Acetyl Cysteine (NAC)** – a lesser-known nutrient with many benefits. In this instance you should know that it supports the deepest level of your body's ability to neutralize free radicals. That level is called the glutathione antioxidant system.

- **Selenium** – an essential nutrient mineral. Also an excellent antioxidant.

- **Co-Q10** – an enzyme in your cells responsible for generating energy. Also a potent antioxidant. The best form of this is called ubiquinol. If you take this you will probably need to get it separately from an antioxidant formula.

- **L-Carnosine** - a multi-potent super-antioxidant. It protects cell membranes. Although present in the body, levels go down with age.

Note that you can overdo antioxidants. This is definitely a case where a little is enough. There is no point in loading up on high doses. If you are eating whole, fresh organic vegetables and fruits, you are getting a fair number of antioxidants.

## Support Digestion

Since food is the fuel for your metabolism, hopefully you are already eating according to your metabolic needs. But what good is it to eat well if you aren't digesting and making use of your food?

If you are over 30, it makes sense to support your digestion in a number of ways. The first way has to do with digestive enzymes. Your body makes less of these as you age. If you have done your MT testing, then you should have a list of specific enzymes for your unique needs.

If you aren't going to do MT testing, then you should at least be taking digestive enzymes. Usually these will be in the form of a combination of enzymes. Have as many of these as possible in the mix:

- **Protease** – helps digest proteins.

- **Amylase** – helps digest starches.

- **Lipase** – helps digest fats

- **Cellulase** – helps break down cellulose into simple sugars.

- **Lactase** – helps digest milk.

- **Phytase** – releases phosphorus from phytic acid. Phytic acid is in grains and oil seeds and interferes with digestion unless it is converted this way.

- **Maltase** – breaks down maltose, a complex sugar found in some grains.

- **Invertase** – helps your body break down and utilize sucrose (sugar).

- **Galactase** – another enzyme that helps break down milk and milk products.

- **Xylanase** – helps break down cell walls of plant-based foods.

- **Bromelain** – pineapple enzyme, especially good for digesting proteins.

- **Papain** – papaya enzyme, also good for protein digestion.

• **Hemicellulose** – supports complete digestion of cellulose.

## Protect Your Brain

If you've ever seen a loved one go through the misery and frustration of Alzheimer's Disease, then you already understand how important it is to keep your thinking sharp and clear as you age.

Near the end of my Grandmother's life, she experienced this kind of decline. I'd go to visit her and say, "Hi Grandmother, it's your grandson, Bruce," to which she'd often reply, "If you say so…"

Probably because of the aging population of Baby-Boomers, a great deal of research is happening about causes of aging. And much of this research explores the realm of cognitive function.

How well your brain works goes a long way towards supporting quality of life. It's a very good idea to do things that support your brain.

Here's what we know so far about making sure that you'll have the best chance for keeping mentally clear long into your retirement years:

**Exercise**: Physical activity not only supports a healthy body, but also contributes greatly to a healthy mind. And it's never too late to start. Even elderly people who are losing their mental focus can improve by starting a walking program.

**Dietary Fats**: For 40 years we've been told that fat is bad. And truthfully, some fat is. By avoiding trans-fats, most vegetable oils, hydrogenated oils, shortening and other deadly forms of fat, you are helping your body and brain stay healthier.

But your brain also needs healthy fats to function efficiently. The healthiest of these are fish oils, which are high in Omega-3 fatty acids. I can't over-emphasize how important it is to make sure you're getting enough of these essential fats. Two other very beneficial sources of healthy fats are extra virgin olive oil and coconut oil (virgin pressed).

**Antioxidants**: Just as free radicals circulating through your blood stream damage your body, they also damage your brain. Make sure you're eating antioxidant-rich foods and taking supplements high in these important substances.

**Defeat Stress**: It's hard to eliminate stress living in modern times. But doing everything you can to manage it will help you keep your brain strong and healthy. The reason is that stress causes the release of the brain cell damaging hormone, cortisol.

Making time for such activities as meditation, positive mental imagery, yoga, qigong, etc. will help defeat the negative effects of stress.

**Use It or Lose It**: Just like muscles, your brain gets stronger with use. The key to keeping it strong is exposing it to new experiences. Particularly helpful are activities like learning a new language, tackling challenging mental puzzles, reading interesting books and engaging in stimulating conversations.

**Brain Supplements**: There are many supplements that support your brain. Here is a list of the more important ones:

- **Omega 3 Fatty Acids**: You've heard about using fish oil for a variety of health issues, particularly inflammation. Its anti-inflammatory properties are impressive and no doubt support a healthy brain. But one of the components in it (DHA) also demonstrates brain protective activity. In the well-known Framingham Heart Study, participants who had greater intake of DHA had a lower incidence of Alzheimer's disease and other types of dementia, compared with people who consume less DHA.

- **Vinpocetine**: Vinpocetine comes from the periwinkle plant. In Europe they've used this supplement for over two decades to treat cerebro-vascular disorders such as strokes as well as related symptoms. Experiments with vinpocetine indicate that it can dilate blood vessels, enhance circulation in the brain, improve oxygen use, increase red blood cells viability, and prevent sticky platelets. Vinpocetine is also an antioxidant. Some experiments also demonstrate a marked improvement in memory. You should be cautious however when starting this supplement since high doses of vinpocetine can cause the side effect of dizziness, weakness, and uneasy feeling. Although the commonly suggested daily dosage is 10 mg for each 50 pounds of body weight, it's best to be cautious at the beginning. Spread the dose out over the day and avoid taking a 10 mg dosage unless you have first tried half of a 5 mg dose at a time.

- **Alpha GPC (l-alpha-glyceryl-phosphorylcholine)**: GPC gave big improvements in Alzheimer's patients in a multicenter controlled study. It also increased recovery in memory and thinking in post-stroke patients.

- **B-6, B-12, Folic Acid**: These three supplements help reduce the inflammatory substance, homocysteine. Reduced homocysteine levels go along with a dramatically reduced likelihood of a stroke or heart attack as well as decreased memory. You don't need massive doses of these to be effective, but likely more than the government RDA.

- **Acetyl-l Carnitine (ALC)**: Both l-Carnitine and ALC help support energy production in your cells. However, ALC crosses the blood-brain barrier more easily and thus is more specific for increasing available energy in the brain. Studies indicate this translates to improved mood, better memory and clearer thinking.

- **PQQ (Pyrroloquinoline quinone)**: PQQ protects brain cells from toxicity. It also can reverse brain damage caused by chronic oxidative stress. In addition, it supports the creation of new brain cells. Be sure to take the ideal dose, which is 10 mg.

## Support Your Adrenals

Most people's adrenals are not at peak performance. This affects almost every part of their body.

As mentioned before, saliva testing is an excellent way to find out the status of your adrenals. It will also help your practitioner figure out the best way to treat it.

However in lieu of testing, there are some general supplements you can consider:

- **Eleutherococcus (Siberian Ginseng)** – a very strong adaptogen. Supports healthy adrenal function.

- **Panax Ginseng** – good overall tonic, including the adrenals.

- **Astragalus** – brings strength to muscles and supports adaptation.

- **Rhodiola** - effective for supporting weak adrenals.

- Vitamins B-5 (Pantothenic Acid), B-6 (Pyridoxine) and C – all are necessary for healthy adrenal function.

- **Purified adrenal tissue extract** – be sure to get naturally-raised or organic.

When taking adrenal support supplements, it's best to only take them in the morning and at noon. Some people find that they have a somewhat stimulating effect that might interfere with sleep.

## Keep Your Hormones Strong

Keeping your adrenals healthy will go a long way towards good hormone levels. In addition to those mentioned above, there are special herbs that specifically support healthy hormones.

The key to using these is getting them from a quality source. As you might imagine, there are many questionable companies trying to get your dollars for these kind of supplements.

Here are some of the best and rarest:

- **Tongkat Ali** – used for centuries in Sumatra to enhance sexual performance. It has the reputation of letting a man have the same quality sex they enjoyed in youth. Some report their experience is even better than in younger years. And modern research shows that it safely increases testosterone levels. Women can also take it in smaller doses.

- **Deer Antler** – harvested without killing or hurting the animal in any way. When taken, it supports high levels of endurance, preserves youthfulness and enhances longevity. But you only get the benefit when it comes from the very end of the growing tip of the antler. Many sources use more than the tip, diluting the effect. Others don't even include the tip since it is more expensive.

- **Polyrachous Ant** – supports physical stamina and staying power. Chinese Emperors had dozens, and sometimes hundreds of concubines. And they used this to improve their endurance. Because of this it gained the nickname "The Herb of Kings."

# 6. PUTTING IT ALL TOGETHER – THE PERFECT PROGRAM

By now you know that there are steps you can take to upgrade your health. You have also seen that there are three general areas to pay attention to.

You want to:

1) **Reduce symptoms.**

2) **Correct underlying causes of symptoms.**

3) **Repair damage and rebuild health.**

There is a lot of good information about this in the previous chapters. I use this approach with my Executive Health Upgrade patients.

But since there is so much information, you might be wondering how you can make effective use of it. That's what this chapter is about.

Before talking about the "perfect" program, you should keep in mind that what is perfect for one person won't be perfect for another. Even so, it is possible to design a useful program in general terms. Having this information will save you time and help you focus in on your ideal health upgrade.

When it comes to reducing symptoms, you will find everything you need in Chapter 2. Here in this chapter you will find the outline of an effective way to address underlying causes and rebuild health.

## The First Thing: Know What To Correct

Taking action without knowing your state of health is not efficient. It's a little like getting on a bus without knowing where it is going. You can do it, but it is a hit or miss proposition. Later in this chapter I will offer a good basic program that you can do without testing. But I encourage you to have as much information as you can. That's the way to get the biggest benefits from the Total Health Upgrade Program.

For most of these tests, you will need to have access to a doctor who practices functional medicine. When there are ways to get the testing done on your own, I will mention it. Before running any tests or taking any corrective action, be sure to make note of all medications and prescriptions you are taking. You need to rule out side effects causing symptoms.

To gather the best information about what needs addressing, here is a list of the most important tests:

## Tests You Can Do On Your Own

**Metabolic Typing® (MT)** – This is the only way to determine the ideal foods for your metabolic needs. When you know which are right for you, you can:

- Achieve biochemical balance.

- Maximize metabolic efficiency.

- Restore functional efficiency.

- Produce peak performance.

- Obtain optimal health.

- Unfold full genetic potential.

The test is done using an extensive questionnaire. The best way to get this done is through Certified Metabolic Typing® Advisor. Next best is to use the do-it-yourself online test. You can find that test here: www.MetabolicTypingOnline.com.

The disadvantage of doing it yourself is that you won't have access to advanced material. You also won't have someone who can take you through the process, answer questions, etc.

**Cellular Inflammation Test** – There are two types of inflammation. The first is the common redness, pain and swelling from injury. The second is in your cells. This second type doesn't have pain, but it does disrupt hormonal signaling networks throughout the body. It is possible to do this test on your own. The results come with simple guidelines to correct inflammation. The web site is here: http://zonediagnostics.com.

## Tests That Require a Professional

**Hair Tissue Mineral Analysis** – Finds deep mineral imbalances as well as toxic heavy metal exposure. Tests for 36 elements. This test is done by taking a small sample of hair, usually from your head.

**Metabolic Profile Test** – Identifies problem areas to address:

- Detoxification efficiency.

- Digestive efficiency.

- Oxidative stress.

Once you know how each of these systems are working, you can either make corrections, or else have a clear idea of what additional tests should be run.

**Environmental Pollutants Panel** – Measures the presence of 11 environmental toxins in your body. Most people are very surprised at how many they have. Sets the stage, along with the Hair Tissue Mineral Analysis for focused detoxification. Once toxins are addressed, your body functions at a much higher level.

**Steroidal Hormone Balance Test** – This is also called an Adrenal Stress Profile. Because your adrenals are your organs of survival, it is crucial that they work well. This test shows you what degree of fatigue is present and sets the stage for correcting the problem.

**Mediator Release Test** – One very common blocking factor affecting health is food intolerance. When you eat foods your body reacts to, it sets up many kinds of potential negative responses.

**Neurotransmitter Test** – Very useful for a variety of issues. Stress, depression, anxiety, sexual problems and low motivation all benefit from this.

## Working with Results

There are other tests that can be done. However not everyone needs every test. These are done on an as-needed basis. Your practitioner will tell you what you need.

Once you have a clear idea of what needs attention, you can take action. For all but the Metabolic Typing® test and the Cellular Inflammation Test, your practitioner will be able to take you through how to fix problems.

However some people resist getting professional help. If that includes you, here is a simplified program that will likely move you closer to optimal health.

## A "No Test" Program for Upgrading Your Health

What if you don't have access to a physician who practices Metabolic Typing® and Functional Medicine? If that's the case, I still recommend you do the Metabolic Typing online test (link above) and the Cellular Inflammation Test. And, of course, I recommend you follow the recommendations you get with the results.

In addition to those, here is a good general program that will help you reach higher levels of health. Here are the steps to take:

**Cut Out Artificial Foods** – many foods fall into this category. Packaged foods, foods in cans, bottles and jars are worth dropping. Also eliminate anything with preservatives, artificial sweeteners, or GMO ingredients. Eating primarily whole, fresh, organic food will go a long way towards meeting this goal.

**Detoxification** – to detoxify from pretty much any toxins you might have been exposed to, D-Toxol is the best remedy available. The list of toxic substances it helps clear is extensive. It includes radiation, EMF's, plastics, rocket fuel residue, BPA, phthalates, hydrocarbons, heavy metals, medications, fluoride, preservatives, aspartame, MSG, pesticides, and many others. Currently, the only place you can get is UltraLife, Inc. at www.ultralifeinc.com.

**General Supplementation** – Most food in modern times lacks nutrients compared to 100 years ago. That makes supplementation crucial. The best supplements for you can only be determined when you know your Metabolic Type®. The results come with specific recommendations for your unique needs.

If you can't or won't do the MT test, at least take a high-quality, food-grade multi-vitamin with minerals.

In addition to specific nutrients, every supplement regimen should include the following:

- **Omega-3 Fatty Acids** – the best source is fish oil. Find one that is molecularly distilled for the highest purity. Take 1 to 2 at each meal.

- **Digestive Enzymes** – to make sure you are getting maximum benefit from your food. If you know your Metabolic Type®, you will get recommendations for specific ones. Otherwise, get a good general enzyme combination. An excellent one is from UltraLife, Inc. It is called Enzigest. 1 to 5 at each meal.

- **Probiotics** – these are the health-supporting bacteria found in yogurt and similar products. Although you can get foods that have them, I still recommend a supplement that has many different strains. A good general one is called Primal Defense.

**Adrenal Support** – It is possible to get very specific if you've had an adrenal stress lab test done. If not, find a supplement with a good array of adaptogens in it. A web search for the phrase, "adrenal support" will turn up a dizzying variety of products. When you find one you like, take it only in the morning and if needed, again before 2:00. Taking these later in the day can sometimes interfere with sleep.

**Filter Your Water** – All municipal water is chlorinated. And some water also carries other toxic materials. That's why it makes sense to filter the water you drink. I recommend using a reverse osmosis filter.

You might also consider filtering your shower water. You can get small, individual filters for your shower head that will take out chlorine and some other toxins.

**Filter Your Air** – Indoor pollution can be as great or greater than outdoor. That's why it makes sense to make sure the air in your home and office is free from toxic substances.

**Reduce Stress** – This is a big topic because stress can happen from at least 12 different sources. All of the previous recommendations will help reduce the stress load on your body.

But stressors aren't only physical. They can also come from other parts of your life.

For example:

- **Emotional Stress** – these include loss or emotional trauma.

- **Cognitive Stress** – another type of stress comes from receiving irrational demands or unfair judgments.

- **Existential Stress** – having no purpose or direction is a major stressor.

There are a number of ways to manage these types of stress. Here are some of the best ones:

- **Exercise** – not only will this improve your physical health, it also improves your mental and emotional health. It does this by helping reduce the tension that stress creates in the body.

- **Hobbies** – getting your focus off day-to-day problems while doing something you enjoy goes a long way towards reducing stress.

- **Meditation / Prayer** – finding meaning and feeling connected to something bigger than yourself vastly improves your quality of life. Along with this comes a great reduction in stress.

As you can see, this list is fairly general. It may be all you need if you are in relatively good health.

However, if you have specific health issues that don't improve from this general approach, it is best to work with someone trained in Functional Medicine. That's the best way to make sure nothing is left out. And if you have chronic health issues, want to reduce or eliminate medications, or if you want better results please consider working with a professional trained in Functional Medicine.

# ABOUT DR. BRUCE EICHELBERGER

Dr. Eichelberger works with executives and professionals from around the country to increase their health and productivity. These high performing people are smart and successful, but want to reach higher performance through upgrading their health. His approach to helping patients can be summed up in one sentence, "Quality of life is everything."

Because of his own health issues early in life, early on he became interested in finding ways to correct health problems naturally. He still actively researches the most effective ways to reach optimal health and performance.

He offers The Total Health Upgrade Program to his patients. It is the premier method of increasing peak performance. You can learn more about the Total Health Upgrade Program on his web site at:

**http://www.ExecutiveHealthUpgrade**

DR. BRUCE EICHELBERGER

# COPYRIGHT AND DISCLAIMER

The author and publishers of this book do not dispense medical advice nor prescribe to the use of any technique or treatment for medical problems without the advice of a medical professional, either directly or indirectly. It is the intention of this book to only offer information of a general nature. Any specific problems should be referred to your doctor.

If you choose to use this information for yourself then the author and publisher assume no responsibility whatsoever.

www.ingramcontent.com/pod-product-compliance
Lightning Source LLC
Chambersburg PA
CBHW070231290526
45789CB00004B/1574